Paleo Diet Cookbook: 57 Quick and Easy Paleo Diet Recipes

By Rebecca Publishing

Disclaimer

All the material contained in this book is provided for informational and educational purposes only. No responsibility can be taken for any outcomes resulting from the use of this material.

While every attempt has been made to provide information that is both accurate and effective, the author does not assume any responsibility for the accuracy or use/misuse of this information.

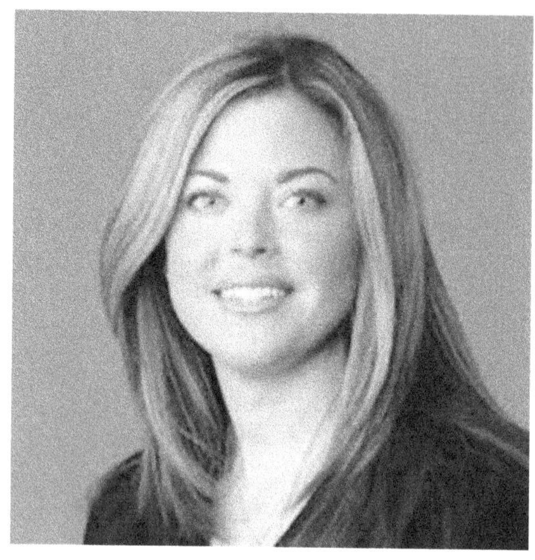

About the author!

I am a newbie to publishing business, but I have a lot of information to tell you. I have been studying healthy way of eating from leading nutritionist in Europe and I have a lot of useful information on this topic. I have lost more than 20 kilos so I can provide you with a lot of practical tips on this matter.

My story is also very bright, after giving birth to a child; I have gained a lot of extra weight. It was simply impossible to look into the mirror, but I decided to do my best to return to my previous shape. I have tried swimming, jogging, different diets like Dukan, Sugar Free Diet, Kremlyovskaya Diet etc. These diets forced me to starving and nothing more. I saw and fell the best result after following the Paleo Diet. This diet helped me to loose ALL my extra weight this is more than 20 kilos/44 pounds and I feel myself much healthier now! So,

I am glad to share with you 57 of my beloved paleo recipes, I hope you will find them healthy and delicious as well.

Introduction

Thank you for downloading of my Paleo Diet Cookbook: 57 Quick and easy Paleo Diet Recipes. All the recipes were tried and prepared by me and they really helped me to loose weight and stay healthy at the same time. I am more than happy to share them with you!

1. ALMOND FLOUR PANCAKES

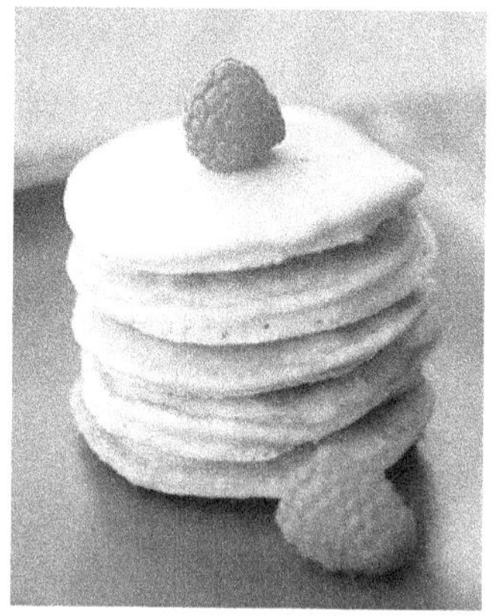

Ingredients:

one and a half cup of almond flour

one and a half cup of apple sauce, no sugar

one tbsp of coconut flour

two large eggs

less than a half of a cup of a water

less than a half of tsp of nutmeg

less than a half of tsp of sea salt

one tsp of coconut oil

half of a cup of fresh berries

Instructions:

1.Put all the ingredients into a bowl, like: almond flour, apple sauce, coconut flour, eggs, water, nutmeg and sea salt.

2. Stir all this together with a fork.

3. Heat the frying pan with coconut oil.

4. Add one fourth of a batter into the pan

5. Flip like a usual pancake when you can see the bubbles and prepare for one more minute.

6. Add some oil and repeat with the remaining batter.

7. Put some fresh berries on the top.

2. APPLE CINNAMON MUFFINS

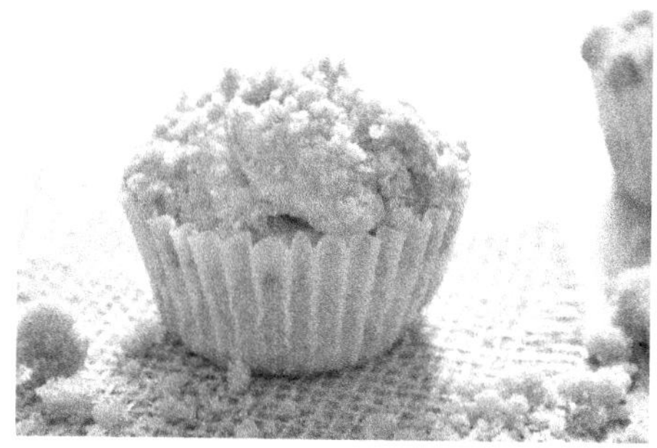

Ingredients:

Two small apples cored and diced

One tbsp. of lemon juice

Five large eggs

A half of a cup of coconut flour

Two tablespoons of cinnamon

A bit of ground nutmeg

One tbsp of baking soda

Four tsp of melted coconut oil

A bit of a sea salt

One package of paper muffin liners

Instructions:

1. Preheat the oven, sprinkle a muffin tin with cooking spray or it is possible just to put paper liners.
2. Put all the apples into the saucepan and cover. It is necessary to add enough water so it will cover almost the half. Wait until it boils and later reduce heat and let it simmer for 10 minutes. You will be sure everything is ready when apples are broken down. Make everything smooth with the help of a blender.

3. Let the apples to cool, when everything is ready, add other ingredients to the blender and puree till the thick batter.

4. Add butter into your muffin tin

5. Bake approximately 15 -18 minutes until muffins get browned. Let them cool before taking out from the pan.

3. BANANA TAPIOCA CREPES

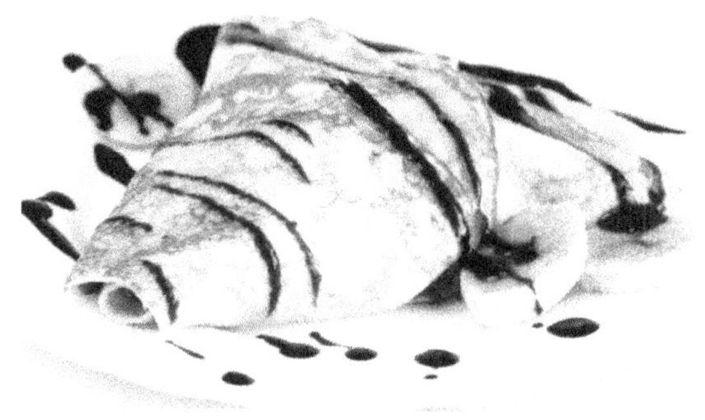

Ingredients:

Seven large eggs

Five large bananas

One can of coconut milk

One tsp of sea salt

Two and a half cups of starch or tapioca flour.

Instructions:

1. Put all the ingredients together and make a soupy butter
2. Preheat the pan
3. When the pan becomes hot add thin layer of batter
4. Cook until both sides are lightly browned.
5. These things are great for wrapping meat and veggies.

4. BERRY COCONUT CHIA SMOOTHIE

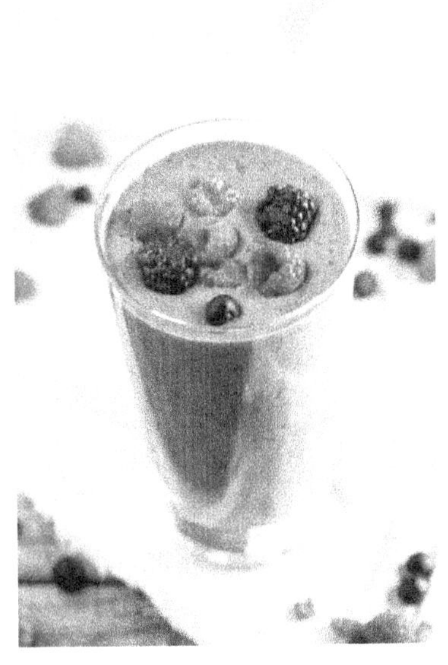

Ingredients:

One medium banana

Two tbsp. of chia seeds

Two cups of spinach baby

One tsp of coconut oil

One and a hald maybe even less of coconut milk, full fat

One cup of frozen berries

One tablespoon of coconut flakes, if you wish to garnish your dish

One tablespoon of chia seeds if you wish to garnish your dish

Instructions:

Put all the stuff into the blan der and blend everything until smooth

5. CARROT BANANA MUFFINS

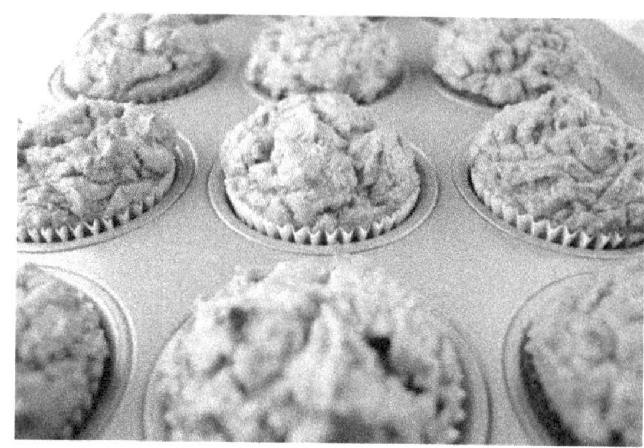

Ingredients:

Two cups of almond flour

Two teaspoons of baking soda

A half of a teaspoon of sea salt

Of tablespoon of cinnamon

One cup of dates

Three medium bananas

Three large eggs

One teaspoon of apple cider vinegar

One fourth of a cup of coconut oil melted

One and a half of a large carrot

A bit of walnuts finely chopped

And paper muffin liners

Instructions:

1. Heat the oven to 350 F.

2. Put together baking soda, salt and cinnamon in a bowl.

3. Add bananas, eggs, vinegar and oil in a food processor.

4. Combine everything plus add carrots and nuts

5. Put this prepared mixture into paper lined muffin tins.

6. Bake for about 30 minutes at 350 F

6. CHORIZO RICE WITH FRIED EGG

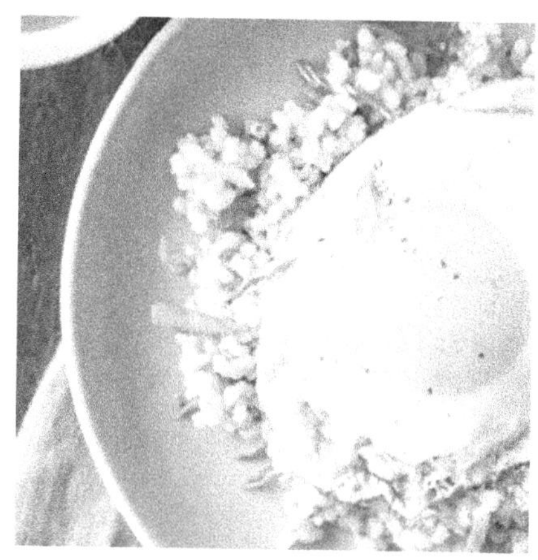

Ingredients:

One pound of ground chorizo

One half of cauliflower

One small onion, diced

One garlic clove , minced

Small bell paper, diced as well

Two eggs

Two tbsp. of a lard

A bit of salt on your taste

A bit of black pepper on your taste

Instructions:

1. You can use a cheese grater to make your cauliflower of a rice like consistency.
2. Heat the pan and add one tbsp. of a lard. Add chorizo and cook for about 7 minutes.
3. Add onion, bell pepper and saute for 1 -2 minutes more.

4. Make the heat lower and add the riced cauliflower to the pan. Cook for another 5 minutes.

5. Also heat up one tablespoon of lard and fry eggs

6. Pile chorizo on a plate and put a fried egg ona top.

7. Garnish with green onions or cilantro if you wish!

7. COCONUT LIME PANCAKES

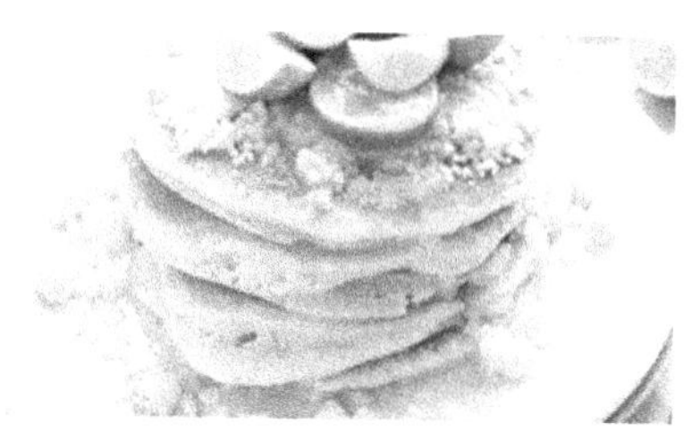

Ingredients:

One and a half cup of coconut, shredded

One and a half of a tsp of baking powder

Salt on your taste

One cup of almond flour

One lime, we need to use its juice

One egg

Two tbsp of honey

One cup of coconut milk

A quarter of a cup of a water

Three tbsp. of coconut oil

Eight tbsp. of maple syrop

Instructions:

1. Heat the oven to 350 F. Put the coconut on the baking sheet and let it to brow for 4 – 5 minutes. After it gets brown put it to a blender jar.

2. Add the baking powder, lime, almond flour and sea salt to blender and blend it for about 5 seconds.

3. Add the lime juice, water, coconut milk, egg and honey in a bowl. Stir everything well. Add all this into the blender and blend all this stuff together. The batter should look pourable. If it is need add one or two tablespoons of water to make the batter thinner.

4. Hit an iron skillet to medium heat. Add the coconut oil and pour the batter into 3 – inch pancakes. Cook it until both sides will be browned.

8. EGG-FREE, GRAIN-FREE PUMPKIN ZUCCHINI MUFFINS

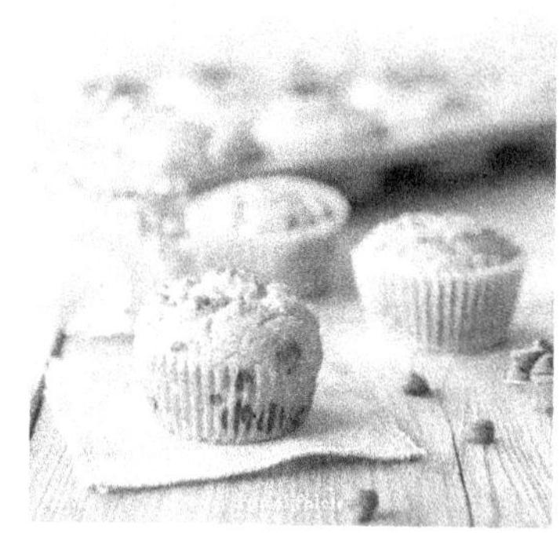

Ingredients:

Two tbsp. of flax seeds

Six tbsp. of water

One cup of almond flour

One and a half cups of coconut flour

One and a half cups of starch

Two teaspoons of baking soda

One tea spoon of sea salt (if you wish)

One tbsp. of cinnamon

One cup of dates

Two cups of pumpkin puree, organic

One tsp of cider vinegar

One spoon of coconut oil

About 10 oz of frozen berries

Grated zucchini ¾ medium

A bit of sliced almonds

One package of paper muffin liners

Instructions:

1. Preheat oven to 350 F.
2. Mix together flax meal and water and let stay for about five minutes.
3. Mix almond flour, coconut flour, tapioca flour, sea salt, cinnamon, baking soda in a large bowl.
4. Put together dates, flax meal mixture, pumpkin, apple cider vinegar and coconut oil in food processor mix everything until dates are totally chopped. Fold into dry ingredients.
5. Add fold berries, nuts and berries into batter.
6. Put into paper lined muffin tins.
7. Bake them for about 20-25 minutes. Than you may turn of the oven and leave the muffins there.

9. FRIED EGGS WITH SWEET POTATO HASH

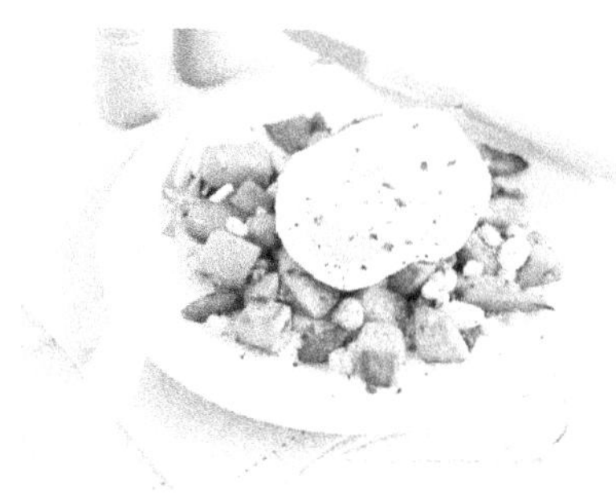

Ingredients:

One tbsp. Coconut oil

One sweet potato, diced into cubes

A half of an onion yellow, diced

Two sausage(s)

One bell pepper, diced

Two tablespoon(s) of water

Four large eggs

A half of a tsp black pepper

Ingredients:

1. Heat coconut oil in a large skillet
2. Satue onions and sweet potatoes for five minutes
3. Add sausages and cook all this together until all the ingredients get browned.
4. Add bell paper and water
5. Cook for about fifteen minutes until the potatoes are totally prepared, stir everything quit often.
6. During all this stuff are being prepared, fry eggs in coconut oil.
7. Season eggs with black pepper and serve all this over sweet potatoe.

10. LIVER SAUSAGE AND EGGS

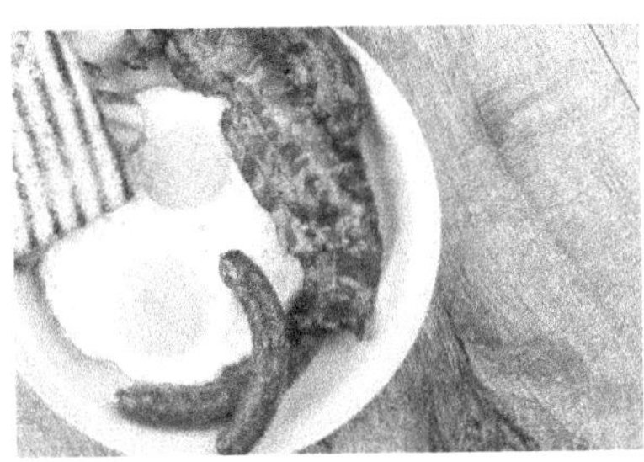

Ingredients:

Three forth pounds of pork

One and a half pound of beef

One forth pound of beef liver

One tsp of maple syrup

One tsp of sage

One and a half of dried thyme

One and a half of tsp of dried rosemary

One and a half of tsp of dried rosemary, sea salt, black pepper

Two tbsp. of olive oil

4 eggs.

Instructions:

1. Put together pork, beef, liver, maple syrup, seasonings, salt, pepper in a bowl. Mix everything thoroughly and form into two-inch patties.

2. Heat the olive oil in a skillet and cook these two patties until well browned. Remove the sausages, add the oil and fried the eggs. Serve with sausages.

11. PUMPKIN BREAD

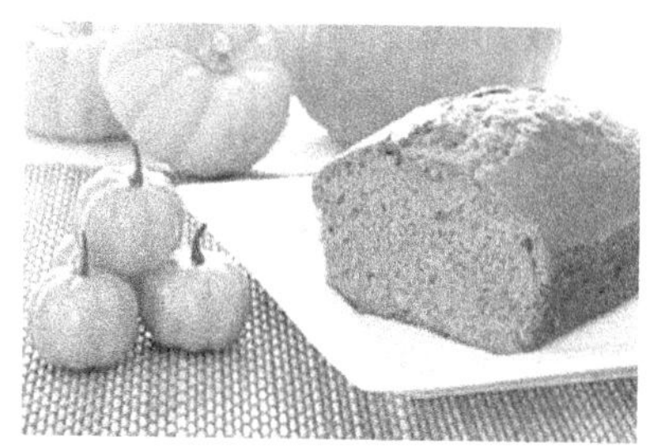

Ingredients:

One cup almond flour

a half of a cup of coconut flour

one Tsp of cinnamon

½ tsp baking soda

½ tsp sea salt, fine grain

½ teaspoon pumpkin pie spice

$1/4$ teaspoon cloves

1 cup coconut sugar

½ cup pumpkin puree,

$1/3$ cup   coconut oil, melted

3 tbsp coconut milk

1 whole vanilla beans

4 large eggs

Instructions:

1. Preheat the oven to 325 F

2. Mix together the flours, cinnamon, salt, pumpkin pie spice, baking soda, cloves, and coconut sugar in the bowl of a large food processor. Then add the pumpkin puree, coconut oil, vanilla bean seeds, coconut milk, or extract, and eggs and process for 30 seconds.

3. Put the mixture to the parchment-lined loaf pan. Bake for 70 to 75 minutes. Let cool in the pan for fifteen minutes.

12. ROASTED PEPPER AND SAUSAGE OMELET

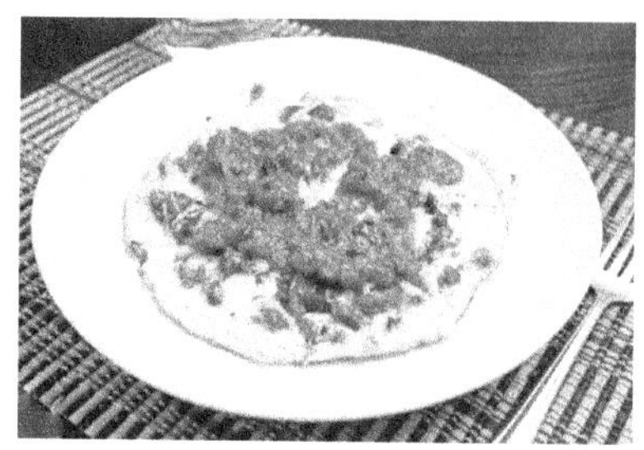

Ingredients:

One green chili or bell pepper.

Four eggs

A bit of a black pepper

2 tsp of coconut oil

One and a half pounds of Italian sausages or you can take beef, cook and slice it

2 tbsp of parsley

Instructions:

1. Put pepper into a pan with a heavy bottom. Make pepper`s skin blacken and blister. When the pepper is ready, remove from the pan and put it into plastic bag, you may add a few drops of water. Wait for 5 more minutes, remove from this bag, cut out seeds, peel the skin and dice.
2. After, beat eggs in a bowl and add black pepper.
3. Heat a skillet over medium heat. Add one tsp of coconut oil when hot.
4. Add half of the egg mixture to preheated pan. As the egg starts preparing, add another half of the remaining ingredients to one half of the pan.
5. When all is set, put half of the egg over the filling, and cook for another minute.
6. Do the same with the second omelet.

13. SUMMER VEGETABLE FRITTAT

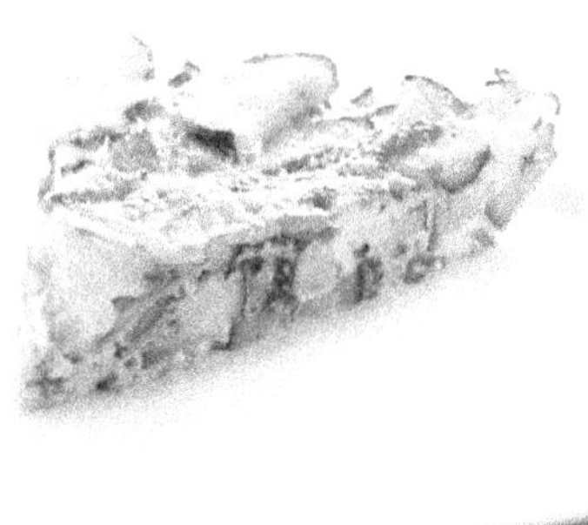

Ingredients:

One and a half tbsp. coconut oil or olive oil

One zucchini

One and a half bell pepper

One and a half onion, Diced

One tablespoon thyme

Sea salt on your taste

Black pepper on your taste

2 garlic cloves, minced

One tomato seeded

9 eggs

Instructions:

1. Heat coconut oil in a oven over medium heat. Add zucchini, pepper, onion, and half of the sea salt, thyme, garlic and pepper.

2. Cover and cook until vegetables are done (it may take you five – seven minutes), stir from time to time.

3. Add tomato. Cook for five more minutes.

4. Mix eggs and salt and pepper.

5. Pour eggs over vegetable mixture and stir everything. Lower heat and cook fifteen more minutes.

6. Put on a plate, slice and serve.

14. WESTERN OMELET

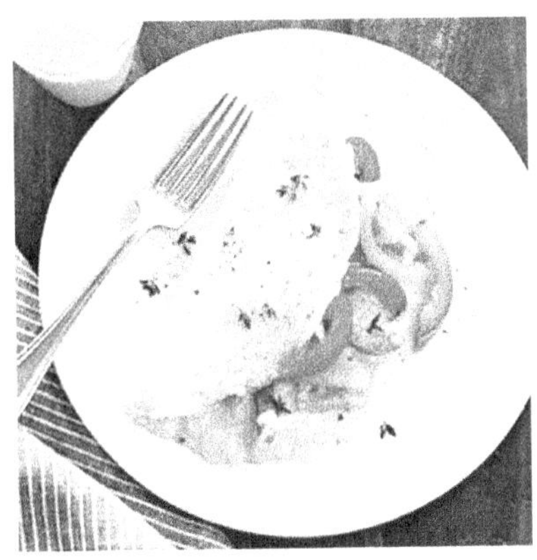

Ingredients:

Four large eggs

One tps of coconut oil

One and a half medium onion

One medium bell pepper

One tomato

One cup of spinach

One forth pounds of ham, cooked and diced

One forth tsp of salt

One forth tsp of black pepper

Instructions:

1. Wash and cut vegetables.

2. Put eggs into small pan and mix well.

3. Heat the skillet. When hot, add coconut oil to the pan.

4. Add half of the beaten eggs into the skillet. When the egg is almost cooked make it pour all over the pan you can help to do it with the fork.

5. Then, add half of the vegetables and ham to the omelet and proceed with the cooking process until the egg is almost prepared.

6. Using a spatula, fold the empty half over top of the ham and veggies. Cook for additional two minutes.

7. The second omelet make in the same way.

15. Veggie & Duck Egg Paleo Breakfast Muffins

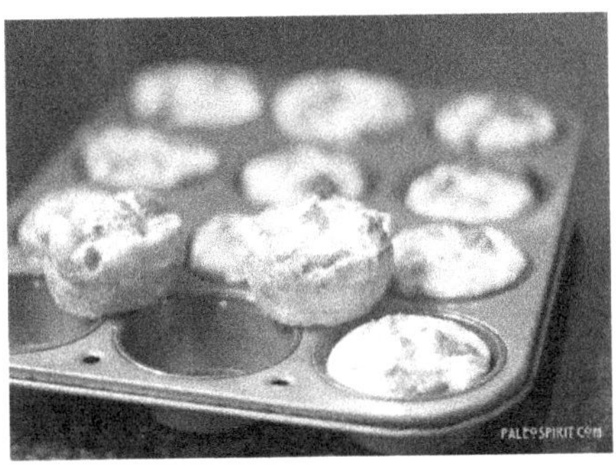

Ingredients:

1 and a half cups of eggplant, diced

Two diced mushrooms

Six tbsp. of tomato sauce

Six duck eggs

Savory leaves dried, according to your taste

Sea salt according to your taste as well

Instructions:

Preheat the oven to 350 F

Fill the muffin tin with parchment paper baking cups.

Fill these muffin cups with diced eggplant and mushrooms.

Add a teaspoon of homemade tomato sauce on top

Cracj a duck egg on top of the sauce

Put on the top of each muffin savory and some salt.

Put the muffin tin into the oven and cook for 15 minutes

Enjoy your meal!

16. Paleo Banana Nut Muffins

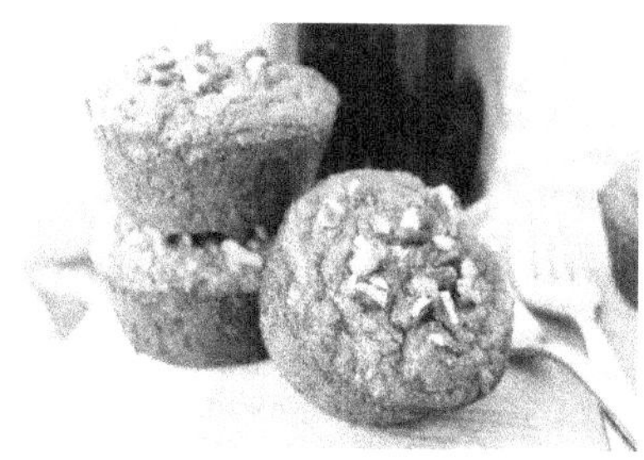

Ingredients:

Two brown bananas

One and one forth cup of an almond flour

One forth cup of tapioca flour

One tsp of baking soda

Three eggs

A bit of raw walnuts

Two tbsp. of lard

A bit of sea salt on your taste

Two tbsp. of honey

Instructions:

1. Heat the oven to 350 F
2. Peel the bananas and put them into the medium-sized bowl.
3. Also add the almond flour, tapioca flour and some baking soda to the bowl with bananas. Stir everything carefully.
4. Bake it for about thirty minutes
5. You can serve it either warm or cold.
6. Enjoy your meal.

17. Paleo Baked Avocado Fries Recipe

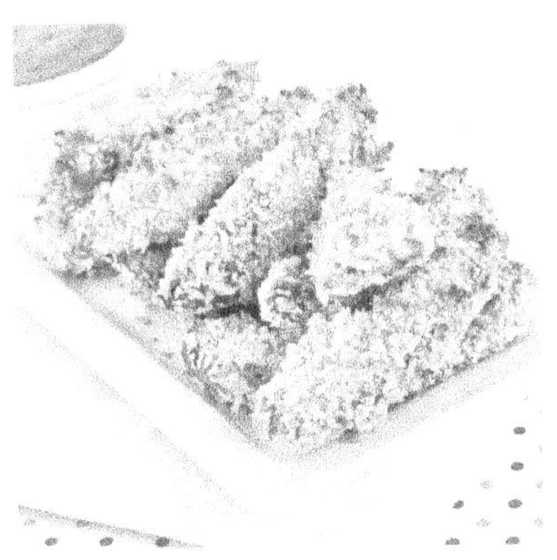

Ingredients:

two avocados

two tea spoon of garlic powder

one tea spoon of onion powder

1 tea spoon of paprika

sea salt on your taste

black pepper on your taste

about 50 g of tapioca flour

one egg

about 15 ml of water

a bit of a stone ground mastered

about 30 g of crushed pork rinds

Instructions:

1. Heat the oven to 425°F

2. Cut the avocados in pieces. Divide each half into several slices, and set them aside.

3. You'll use three small bowls. Mix the arrowroot and half the seasonings into the first bowl. Beat the egg, water and mustard in the second bowl. Put the pork rinds and the other half of the seasonings into the third bowl.

4. After dip the avocado slices into the arrowroot, the next step is eggs, and after the pork rinds. Put everything on the baking sheet. Bake the avocado fries for about fifteen minutes, then turn and toss and bake for another 2 to 4 minutes.

18. Chocolate Collagen Protein Pancakes Recipe

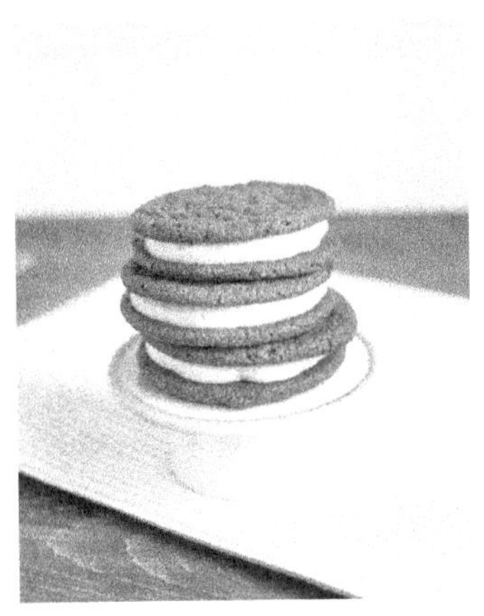

Ingredients:

One egg

Less than a half of almond milk

A half of a cup of a water

One table spoon of honey

Two table spoon of coconut oil

A bit of an almond meal

One forth cup of tapioca starch

Three tea spoon of baking powder

Three table spoon of cacao powder

One forth cup of collagen powder

A bit of salt on your taste

You can also add some fresh fruits

You can put some honey on top if you like

Instructions:

Mix egg, water and almond milk in a bowl. After that add coconut oil and honey and mix everything thoroughly.

Mix almond meal, baking powder, salt, cocoa powder, tapioca starch and collagen in another bowl.

It is necessary to get a thick batter by joining together dry ingredients together with the wet ingredients by whisking them thoroughly.

Heat the coconut oil in the prepared skillet and put in the middle of it in the form of circle.

When you see the bubbles on the top of the batter turn it over with the help of spatula and cook for another minute.

It is even more delicious to serve the pancakes with honey or fruits on the top.

19. Basic Chestnut Flour Crepes

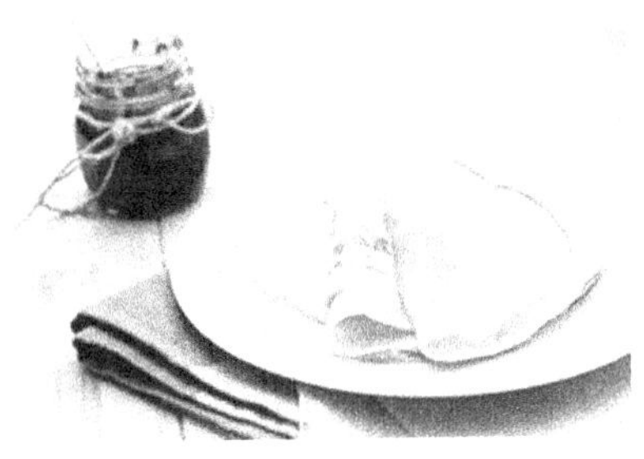

Ingredients:

Two cups of chestnut flour

One cup of milk

one cup of water

one egg

one tbsp. of coconut oil

Instructions:

1. Mix milk, water, and egg in a blender.
2. Add two hundred grams of chestnut flour in a blender
3. Add some melted butter it also can be oil.
4. Mix everything for five ten minutes.
5. Heat a skillet.
6. Pour the batter about one third of a cup into pan. Cook it until you see that the surface is no longer raw and you can see that the other side is already brown. If it is so than flip it on the other to make it golden.

Snack Recipes

20. ALMOND MUFFINS

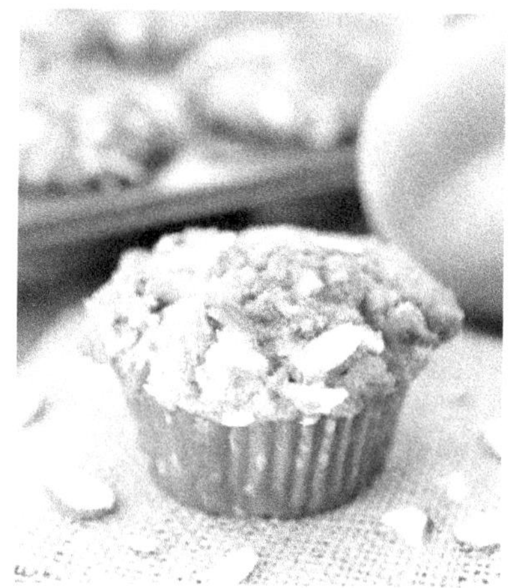

Ingredients:

One cup of almond butter

One cup of almonds

One cup of coconut milk

Two cups of coconut

Three large eggs

A bit of vanilla

Two tbsp. of honey (if you like it)

One package of muffin liners

Instructions:

Heat the oven to 400F

Line a tin with the necessary paper

Mix together all the ingredients and put into the muffin tin.

Bake for about twenty minutes.

21. BACON AND TOMATO SWEET POTATO

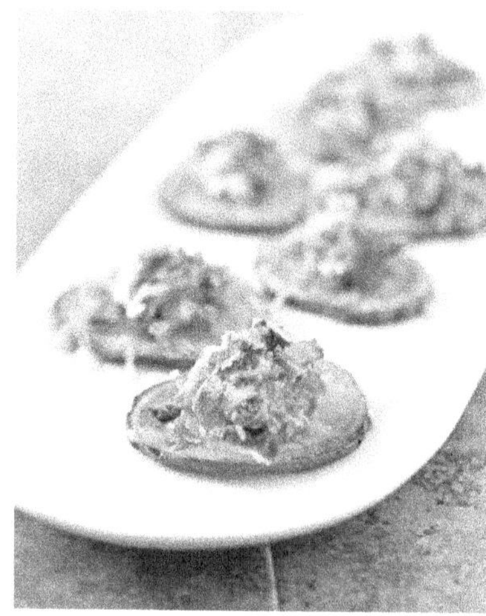

Ingredients:

Two sweet potato

Two tbsp. of olive oil

Two cups of cherry or grape or tomatoes can fit as well. It is necessary to cut into quarters.

Six slices of a bacon, it is necessary to cook it and make crispy

A bit of a freshly chopped parsley

A bit of a sea salt on your taste

A bit of a black pepper on your taste

Instructions:
1. Put a special pepper on a baking sheet, also preheat the broiler. Cut the sweet potatoes and put it onto the baking sheet.
2. Sprinkle with olive oil and salt. Broil until it is cooked.
3. Mix together the tomatoes and the cooked bacon add parsley. Add fresh ground pepper and also put the slices onto the sweet potato before serving.

22. BLUEBERRY COCONUT CEREALS

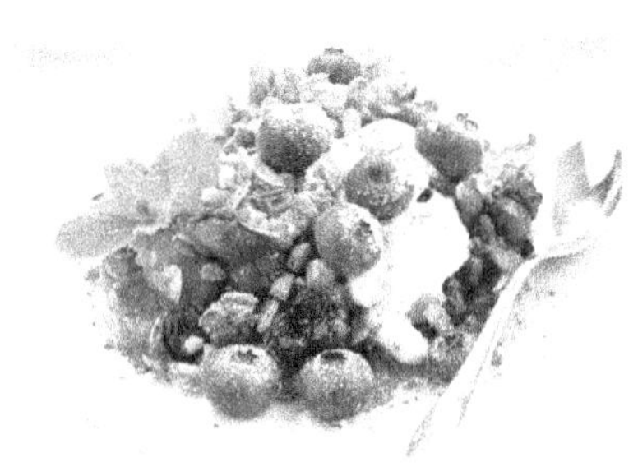

Ingredients:

two cups of chopped pecans

one third cup of coconut oil

six or seven dates

one cup of pumpkin seeds

one tbsp. of vanilla

two tbsp. of cinnamon

a half of tsp of sea salt

one half of coconut flakes, unsweetened

one half of blueberries

Instructions:

1.   Heat the oven to 325F.
2.   Put pecans, coconut oil, dates in a food processor. Mix everything up thoroughly
3.   Add the pecans and pumpkin seeds and ground everything thoroughly as well.
4.   Put to a bowl and put some vanilla, cinnamon and salt. Stir and spread on a baking sheet.
5.   Bake for approximately twenty minutes, until browned. Take away, let them cool, and stir in the coconut and blueberries.

23. CHOCOLATE COCONUT DROPS

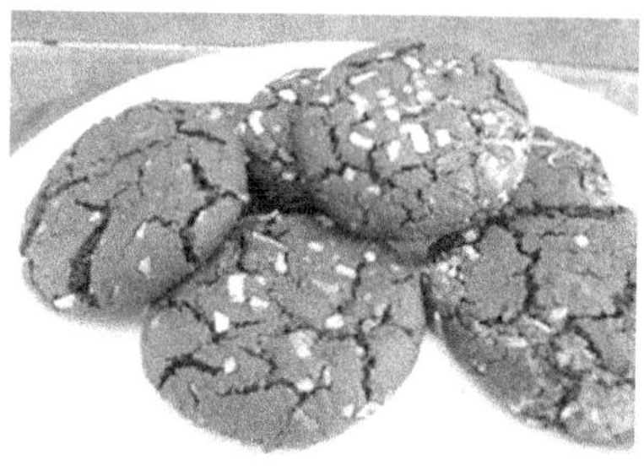

Ingredients:

three tbsp. of coconut oil

one and a half of dark chocolate chips

one and a half of cocoa powder

two tbsp. of honey

less than a half of almond butter

one cup of coconut flakes

Instructions:

1. Put the chocolate chips and coconut oil in the microwave. Cook in thirty minutes intervals until you see that the chips are melted.
2. Put the coconut oil and chocolate chips in a microwave safe bowl. Cook in 30 second intervals until chips are melted, stirring between each interval.
3. Stir all the cocoa powder plus honey, and almond butter. When everything is smooth, add the coconut and stir until well perfectly.
4. Put a baking sheet with special. Put into the fridge until cookies are steady.

24. MINI FLOURLESS CHOCOLATE CAKES

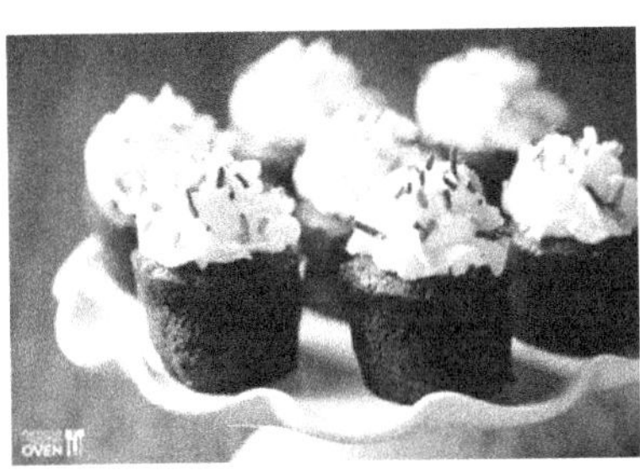

Ingredients:

Two bananas;

One egg;

Two table spoon of honey;

four table spoon of dark cocoa powder;

vanilla on the edge of a spoon

two table spoons of sliced almonds;

Instructions:

Heat the oven to 375 F.

Stir together all ingredients using the blender

Pour the liquid into two separate bowls; put almonds on the top.

Bake for twenty - five minutes approximately.

25. PUMPKIN COOKIES

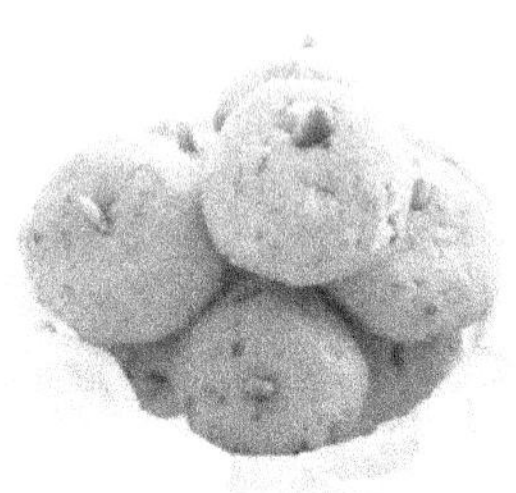

Ingredients:

One cup of pumpkin puree;

Less than a half of a cup applesauce;

Less than a half of coconut milk

One teaspoon of vanilla

one cup of almond meal;

a half of a cup of coconut flour;

a half of a tea spoon of pumpkin pie spice;

Instructions:

Heat the oven to 350 F.

Put the applesauce, coconut milk, pumpkin puree, coconut milk in a bowl. Mix everything well.

Then add the coconut flour and almond meal and stir everything well as well.

On a baking sheet put the parchment and put the batter on it with the help of a spoon.

Place the baking sheet in the oven and leave it there for thirty minutes or so.

26. PALEO GRANOLA

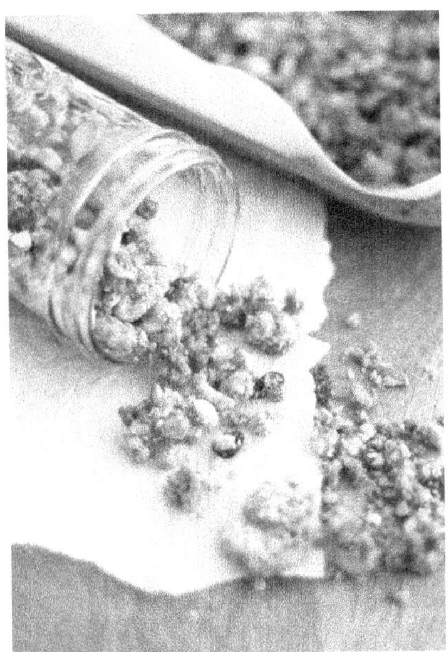

Ingredients:

Raw almonds - 140 g

Raw cashews - 140 g

Raw pumpkin seeds (shelled) - 35 g

Raw sunflower seeds (shelled) - 35 g

Unsweetened coconut flakes - 70 g

Coconut oil - 60 ml

Honey - 120 ml

Powdered vanillin - one tsp.

Sea salt - one tsp.

Raisins (or any dried fruits) - 140 g

Instructions:

1. Heat the oven to 135 C in advance.

2. Grind seeds, almonds, cashews in a blender for several minutes.

3. Mix soft butter, coconut oil, honey and powered vanilla in a medium sized saucepan. Let all components melt over medium-high heat.

4. Add the ground nut mixture and stir well.

5. Take a baking sheet, line it with permanent paper and pour the granola mixture.

6 Do brown during 20-25 minutes.

7. Take finished granola out of the oven. Spread the raisins or dried fruits and sea salt.

8. Press the mixture together. Form a flat, tight surface.

9. Cool for about 20-30 minutes. Cut into and chunks.

10. You may store granola in an sealed container for about a week.

27. PALEO NUT ENERGY BARS

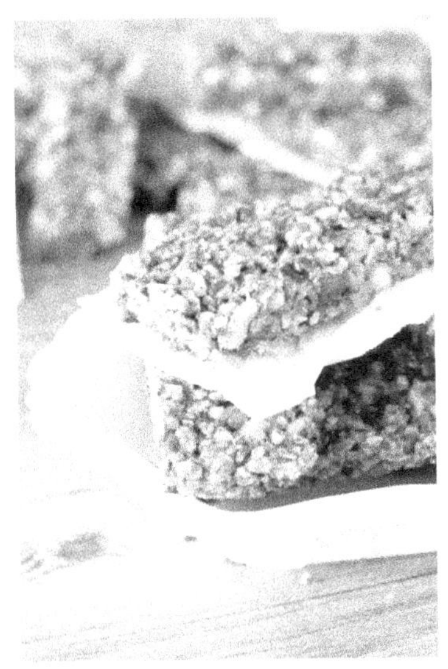

Ingredients:

Chopped pecans - 200 g

Chopped walnuts - 100 g

Chopped almonds - 100 g

Dates - 20 pcs

Liquid egg whites - 250 g

Cinnamon - two tblsp.

Powdered vanillin - 1,5 tsp

Instructions:

1. Preheat the oven to 175 C.

2. Take a large cup and combine all components.

3. Prepare the dish for baking. Line it with pergament paper or aluminum leaf and oil it. Pour out the nut mixture on a dish and press well.

4. Bake for about fifteen-sixteen minutes.

5. Remove energy nut bars from the oven.

6. Let them to get cool for five minutes.

6. Slice the bars.

7. Enjoy bars and energize for the whole day!

28. Homemade Strawberry Fruit Leather

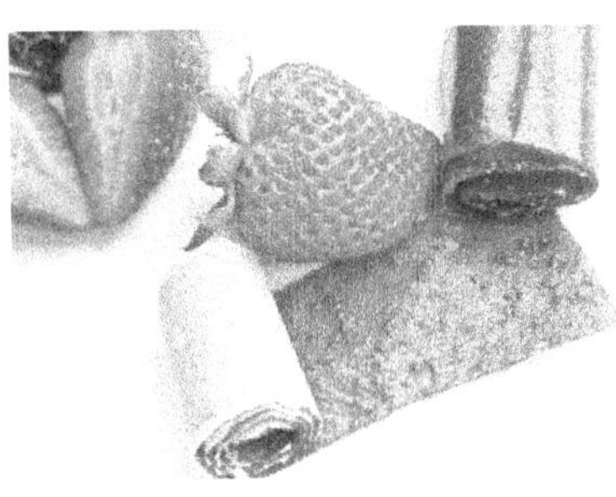

Ingredients:

Chopped strawberries – 400 g

Honey - two tbsp.

Instructions:

1. Heat the oven to 80 C.

2. Put a silpat mat on the baking sheet. Spread berries in a pan and bake at 80 C until soft. Fold in two tablespoons of   honey and stir well.

3. Puree the strawberries   until smooth.

4. Pour honey-strawberries mixture onto the silpat baking mat.

5. Do not raise the temperature and bake for 6 7 hours.

6. When strawberry leather is ready, it should peel away from the silpat mat.

7. Take a knife or scissors to cut this yummy leather into strips.

8. Make rolls to serve!

9. You may store fruit leather in a hermetically sealed package or container.

Paleo Breakfast recipes

29. WEEKEND WARRIOR OMELETTE

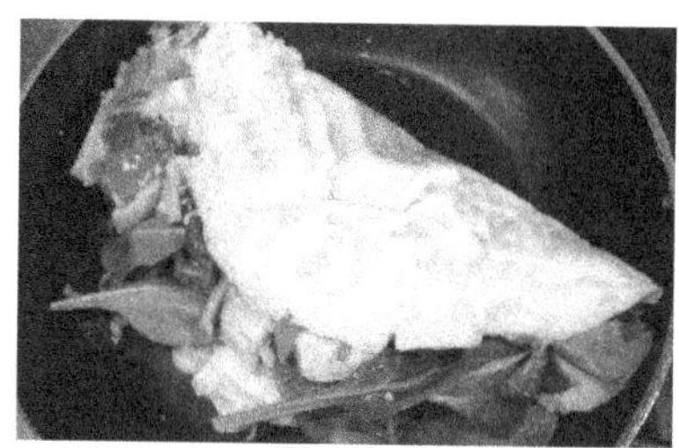

Ingredients:

Organic eggs – 2 pcs

Olive oil - 1 tsp

Green onions – 2 pcs

Organic spinach leaves – 6 pcs

Organic tomatoes – 2 pcs

Half an organic avocado

Instructions:

1. Heat olive oil in a shallow pan.

2. Dice onions and sauté it for 5 minutes.

3. Scramble eggs and pour to onion.

4. Fry for about two minutes.

4. Add diced avocado, tomatoes and salt to taste.

5. Fold in half and turn over Mellette until it fully cooked.

6. Put the scrambled eggs on spinach leaves

7. Enjoy!

30. ROSEMARY ORANGE DUCK WITH ROASTED VEGETABLES

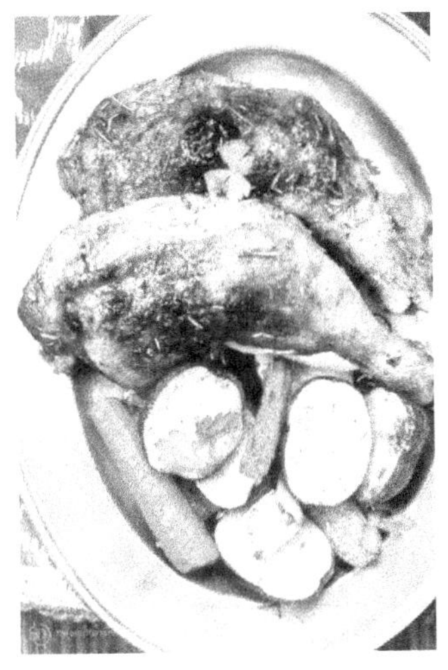

Ingredients:

One big duck

Oranges – two- three pcs

Bunch of rosemary – 1 piece

Carrot – 5-6 pcs

Pasternak – 5-6 pcs

Leek – 3 pcs

Garlic bulblet - 3 pcs

Ground black pepper

Instructions:

1. Take three garlic bulblets, peel and crush them. Wash, peel and chop the carrots and pasternak. Cut three leeks into small rounds.

2. Mix chopped vegetables and add crushed garlic. Thereafter spread this savory blend on the greased bottom of a firepan

3. Take a dressed duck. Wash it and dry with a paper towel. Salt and pepper. If you like, you can slightly spread crushed garlic on the carcass of the duck.

4. Cut two or three oranges into four pieces. Stuff a duck with oranges and rosemary.

5. Put the carcass of the duck on top of the vegetables.

6. Heat the oven to 190 C and place the firepan in it. The duck bakes about three hours.

BUT Every 20 minutes take your duck with vegetables out of the oven to water the juice over it. This helps keep it from drying out.

Three hours later, your rosemary orange duck with roasted vegetables will be ready!

It smells delicious! Taste it!

31. MEMORIAL DAY PALEO GRILLING MARINADES

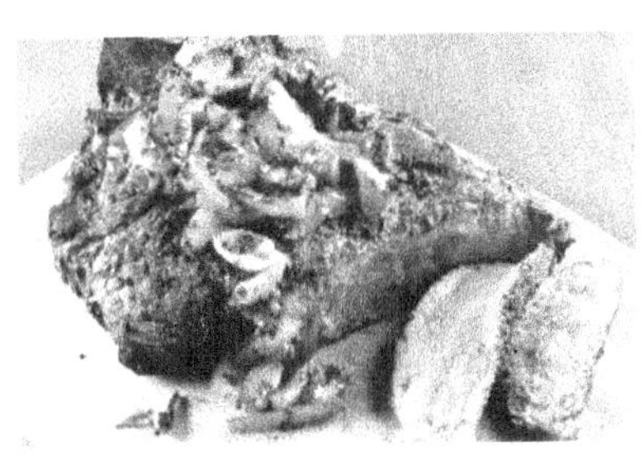

Ingredients:

Melted coconut oil – 1cup

Freshly squeezed Meyer lemon juice – two tbsp

Honey – 1,5 tbsp

A small piece of fresh ginger root

Paprika

Fresh ground black pepper – 0,5 tsp

A pinch of crushed red chili flakes

Garlic bulblet - 5 pcs

Finely chopped spring onion – 3 pcs

Instructions:

1. Take a food processor bowl and put there all ingredients for marinade (except spring onion)

2. Mix thoroughly to reach a homogeneous consistency

3. Spread the marinade on the fish fillet and put into the bowl.

4 The fish is marinated for 30 minutes.

5. Then take it out of the bowl and cook in grill basket.

6. Sprinkle grilled fish with spring onion. Enjoy!

32. SAVORY MEAT

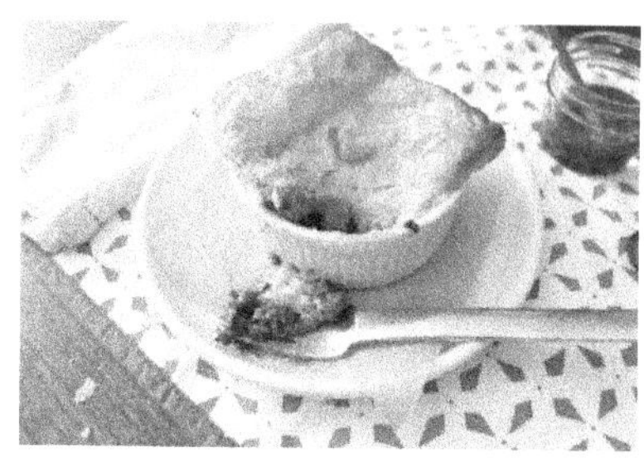

Ingredients:

Freshly squeezed lime juice – 50 ml

Duck fat – three tbsp

Freshly squeezed lemon juice – 15 ml

Ground black pepper

Cumin – one tsp

Garlic bulblet - 4 pcs

Hungarian paprika – one tbsp

Shallot – 2 pcs

Thyme – one tsp.

Instructions:

1. Take a food processor bowl and put there all ingredients. Mix thoroughly to reach a homogeneous consistency.

2. Choose any grass fed meat you like (beet, chicken, goat, turkey etc)

3. Marinade the meat.

4. The meat is marinated for one day

5. Prepare any way you like!

33. SWEET SAVORY MEAT

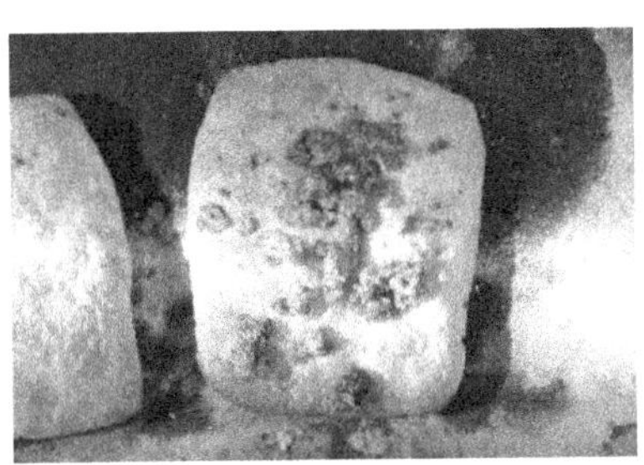

Ingredients:

Orange – 1 piece

Orange zest – one tsp

Melted coconut oil – one cup

Oregano – one tbsp

Freshly squeezed lime juice – 2-3 tbsp

Jalapeno – one piece, seeds removed*

Garlic bulbet – two pcs

Fresh cilantro leaves - 1/2 cup

Instructions:

1. Take a food processor bowl and put there all ingredients. Mix thoroughly to reach a homogeneous consistency.

2. Choose any grass fed meat you like (beet, chicken, goat, turkey etc)

3. Spread the marinade on the meat and put into the bowl.

4. The meat is marinated for one day

5. Prepare any way you like!

PALEO DINNER RECIPES

34. PIZZA SOUP

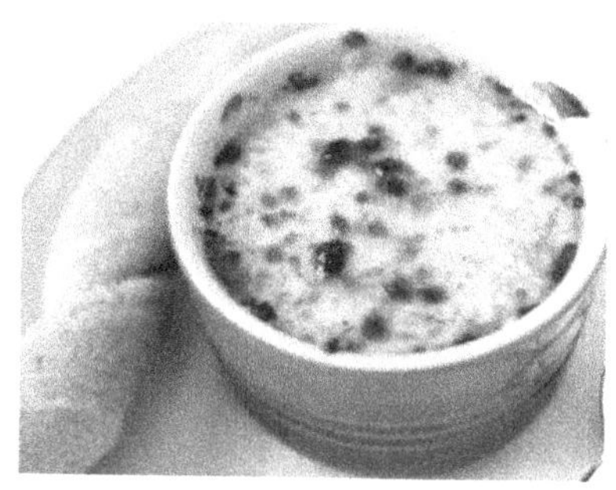

Ingredients:

Sliced chicken sausage – 340 g

Marinara – one jar (700g)

Pepperoni – 115 g (cut into four pieces)

Fire roasted tomatoes – one can (400 g)

Onion – one piece

Sliced mushrooms – 450 g

Sliced black olives – one can (370 g)

Dried oregano – one tbsp

Powdered garlic – one tsp

Salt – 0,5 tsp

Instructions:

1. Take a deep, large saucepan. Put sliced chicken sausage, pepperoni, marinara, one can of fire roasted tomatoes, onion, sliced mushrooms, black olives, one tablespoon of dried oregano, one teaspoon of powdered garlic and salt.

2. Boil over low heat for 30 minutes. Mushrooms and onion should be soft.

3. Add salt if necessary.

4. Your pizza soup is ready!

5. Serve hot!

35. Easy Sweet and Sour Pork

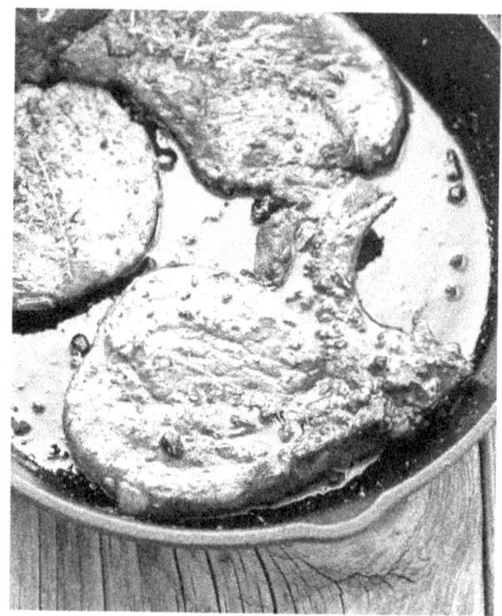

Ingredients:

Bone-in pork chops (225 g each) – four pcs

Butte – two tbspr

Ground black pepper

Salt – one tsp

Balsamic vinegar – two tbsp

Honey - two tbsp

Chopped garlic bulbet – two pcs

Dried rosemary – 0,5 tsp

Dried oregano – 0,5 tsp

Red pepper flakes

Instructions:

1. Heat oven to 200°C.

2. Salt and pepper pork chops. Let marinade.

3. Take the required amount of butter. Melt it on a slow fire.

4. Place pork chops and fry on both sides until browned (2 min per side).

5. Transfer the pan in the oven.

6. Roast for about six minutes.

GLAZE

1. Take a bowl and mix components for glaze.

2. Transfer this spicy mixture into the saucepan. Let it cook slowly (about 5 min).

Back to the chops

1. Remove browned roasted chops from the oven, pour spicy glaze over the top. Back in the oven.

2. Bake for four-five min until caramelized.

3. Serve hot!

36. Spicy Tuna and Tomato Burgers

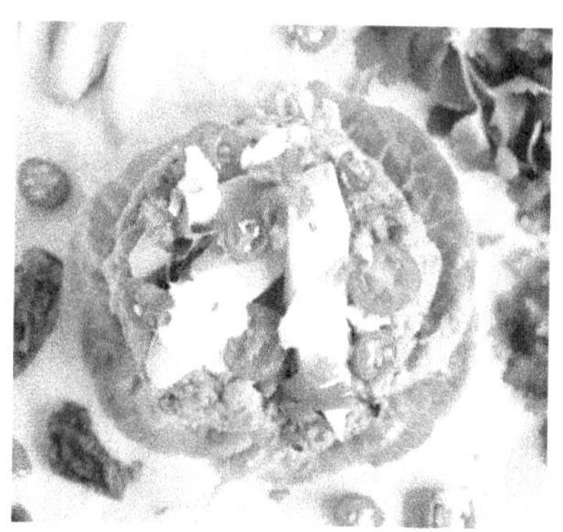

Ingredients:

Tuna – (1x 95g can)

Red onion – one piece

Red chilli – one small piece

Garlic bulbet – one piece

Egg - one piece

Tomato paste – two tbsps

Coconut flour – one tbsp

Salt and pepper

Fresh coriander

Lettuce leaves

Avocado

Sour cream (or Greek yoghurt)

Instructions:

1. Heat the oven to 175'C

2. Use wax paper to line a baking tray.

3. Drain and rinse tuna, chop red onion and red chili, crush garlic bulbets.

4. Toss to combine all ingredients for burger in a bowl.

5. Divide tuna mass into six small sized burgers and put onto prepared baking tray.

6. Place the tray in the oven. Bake for 10 mins, until ready.

7. Serve with fresh juicy lettuce leaves, sliced avocado, add one tbsp of   sour cream (or greek yoghurt) and drizzle with some fresh coriander, salt, pepper and slices of red chilli.

8. Enjoy!

37. Tomato Basil Cauliflower Rice

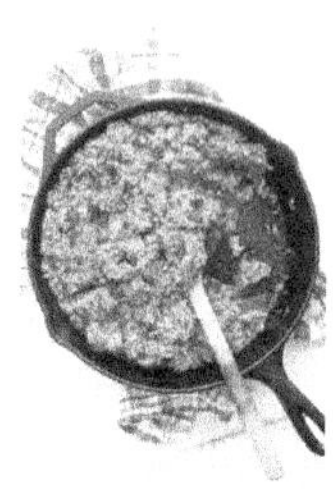

Ingredients:

Cauliflower – one head

Dried Oregano one tsp

Dried Basil – 1,5 tsp

Marjoram – 0,5 tsp

Powdered onion – 0,5 tsp

Chopped garlic – 0,5 tsp

Black pepper

Unsalted tomato paste – 85 g

Dried parsley

Instructions:

1. Divide cauliflower into small curds. Grind in a food processor
2. Take a deep stewing pan and put there the cauliflower and the rest of the components. Stew gently for a further 5-8 mins
3. Remove and serve!

38. Chicken with Cauliflower and Olives

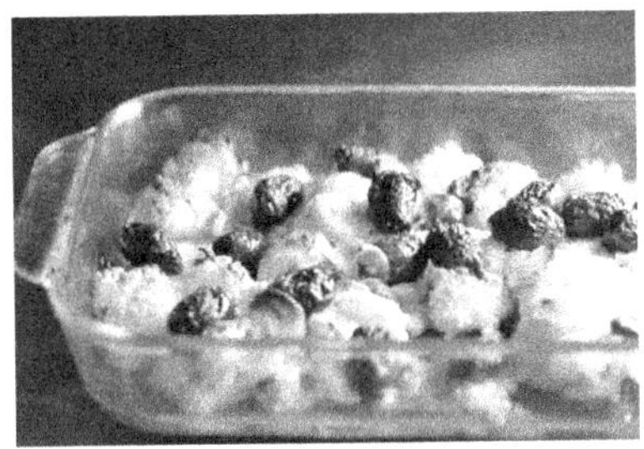

Ingredients:

Chicken breast – 450 g (boneless, skinless)

Thyme sprigs – 1 bunch

Cauliflower – one head (divide into curds)

Shallot – 1 piece

Olive oil - 3 tblsp

Sea salt

Black pepper

Zest of one lemon

Fresh lemon juice - ¼ cup

Kalamata olives - 1 cup, pitted

Garlic bulbet – 5 pcs,

Instructions:

1. Wash chicken breast and dry it.

2. Take some thyme sprigs and place in the baking dish

3. Put chicken breast and cauliflower curds over the thyme sprigs.

4. Take a deep bowl to mix finely chopped shallot, pepper, salt, lemon zest, olive oil, juice, pitted olives and thinly sliced garlic

5. Marinate chicken and cauliflower curds in lemon mixture for a day.

6. Bake chicken with cauliflower curds and olives at 200° for one hour until well browned

7. Serve hot!

39. Sesame Salmon Burgers

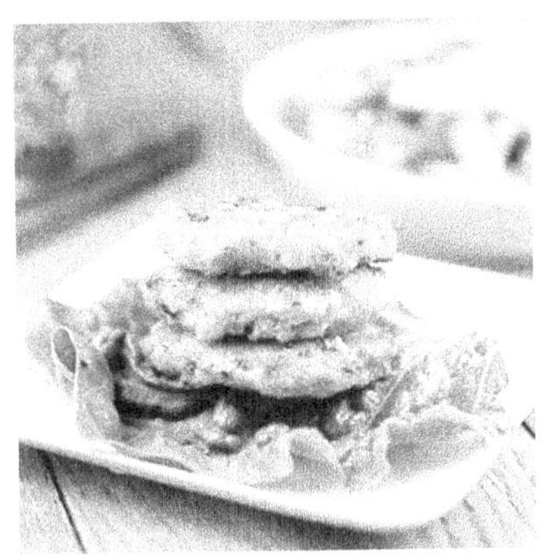

Ingredients:

Salmon - 450 g (skinned)

Egg – 2 pcs

Toasted sesame seeds – 50 g

Toasted sesame oil – 20 ml

Ume plum vinegar – 15 ml

Garlic bulbet - 1 piece (pressed)

Fresh ginger – 5 g (peeled and minced)

Spring onion

Coconut flour – 20 g

Coconut oil

Instructions:

1. Rinse the fish, pat dry and cut into cubes

2. Take a large bowl. Mix toasted sesame oil, ume plum vinegar, pressed garlic, minced ginger, chopped spring onion, toasted sesame seeds and two eggs. Place pieces of salmon in this marinade. Add coconut flour. Stir all ingredients thoroughly.

3. Form small patties.

4. Take a skillet, pour coconut oil in it and heat.

5. Fry the patties until golden brown

6. Put the patties on a paper towel.

7. Serve hot with vegetable puree!

40. Green Chili Turkey Burgers

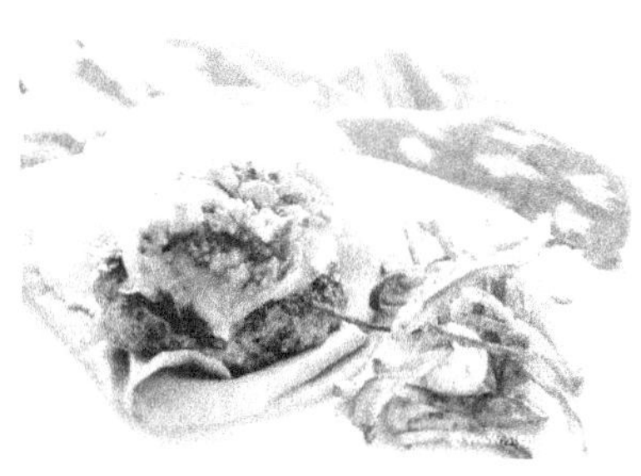

Ingredients:

Diced green chilies (2 cansx112 g)

Ground turkey meat – 450 g

Cilantro – 50 g

Onion – 30 g

Chili powder – 5 g

Cumin – 10 g

Sea salt

Instructions:

1. Prepare a dry big bowl. Put there ground turkey meat and mix with diced green chilies, finely chopped cilantro, onion add salt, chili powder and cumin.

2. Form 8 medium-sized patties and grill them.

3. Serve hot with vegetable puree!

41. Roasted Chicken With Olives And Prunes

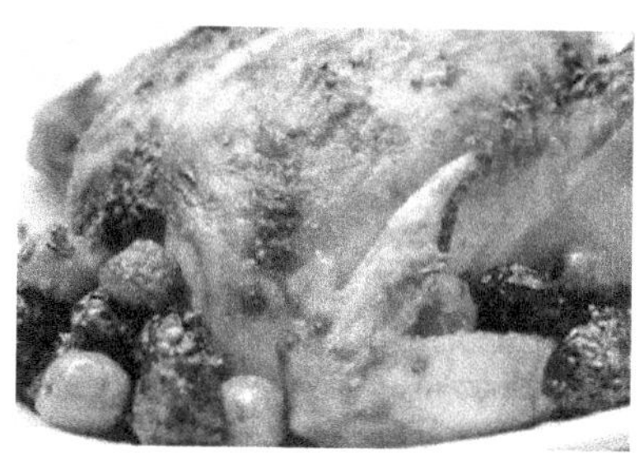

Ingredients:

Dressed chicken – 900-1300 g

Green olives - 150 g (pitted)

Prunes – 150 g (pitted)

Capers – 20 g

Dried oregano – 20 g

Honey – 85 g

Bay leaves – two pcs

Garlic bulbet - 1 piece

Olive oil – 60 ml

Apple vinegar – 60 ml

Water – 60 ml

Sea salt

Instructions:

1. Wash the chicken and pat dry with paper towel.

2. Put the chicken in the baking tray then drizzle with salt

3. Take a large bowl and mix the pitted olives and prunes, 20 g of oregano, 20 g of capers, two flavorous bay leaves, pressed garlic, 60 ml of olive oil and apple vinegar, 60 ml of water. Stir thoroughly.

4. Pour this spicy mixture in the tray around the chicken.

5. Roast the chicken at 220°C for twenty minutes

6. Reduce temperature to 180°C and continue to bake the chicken until until golden crisp (about forty minutes)

7. Take a flavorous, juicy chicken out of the oven and serve.

42. Shrimp Cakes

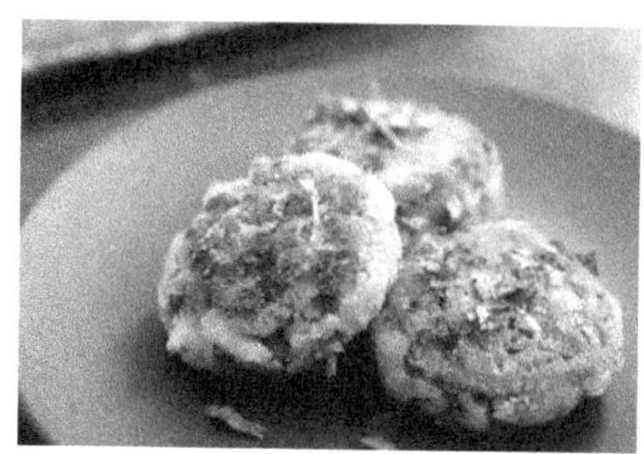

Ingredients:

Raw shrimps – 450 g

Egg – one piece

Blanched almond flour – 60 g

 Red or yellow bell pepper – one piece

Garlic bulbet – 1 piece

 Green onion – two tbsp

Grapeseed oil – 15 ml

Lime juice – 15 ml

Agave nectar – 15 ml

Cilantro – 40 g

Chipotle chile – 2 g

Sea salt

Instructions:

1. Chop raw peeled shrimps in kitchen machine.

2. Take a large bowl and mix chopped shrimps, finely chopped bell pepper, minced garlic, thinly sliced green onion,

15 ml of lime juice, 15 ml of agave nectar, salt, 2 g of chipotle chile, one egg and 40 g of finely chopped cilantro

3. Form 12 thick patties of this mixture and roll in almond flour.

4. Take a large non-stick frying pan, pour 15 ml of oil and heat it.

5. Fry patties on both sides until golden brown (about 5 minutes per side).

6. Line a paper towel on the dish and put the patties on it.

7. Serve with vegetable puree!

43. Curried Prawns

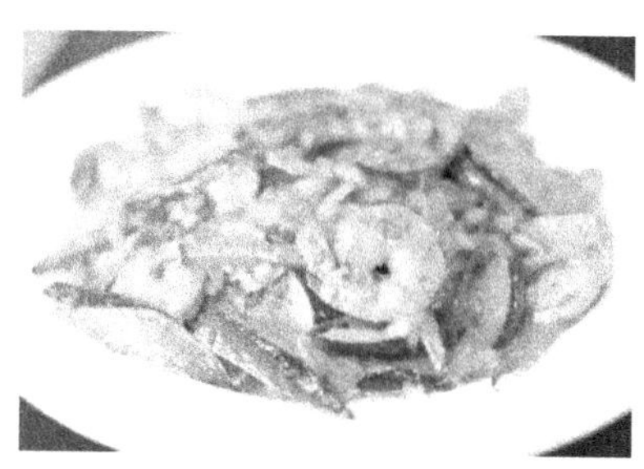

Ingredients:

Large prawns – 450 g

Tomato puree – 120 g

Olive oil – 60 ml

Garlic bulbet – 4 pcs

Onion – 1 piece

Ginger - 40 g

Cumin - ½ tsp

Coriander - ½ tsp

Turmeric -½ tsp

Cilantro -1 bunch

Fresh lime juice – 45 ml

Instructions:

1. Pour olive oil in an enamel pot and heat it.

2. Take peeled and chopped garlic, onion and sauté until tender. Add tomato puree and spices ginger; stew for 5 minutes

3. Put the prawns in the boiling sauce and cook up to readiness (10 minutes).

4. Add finely chopped cilantro. Mix thoroughly.

5. Place on the dish and drizzle with lime juice

44. Lebanese Lemon Chicken

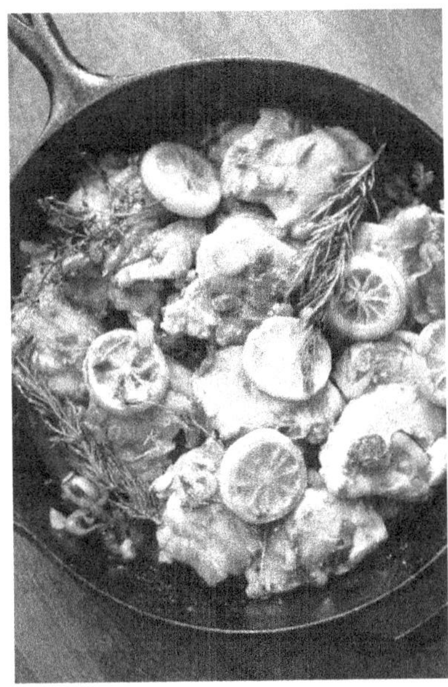

Ingredients:

Chicken thighs – 12 pcs (boneless, skinless)

Olive oil – three tbsp

Organic lemons – three pcs

Lemon – 3 pcs

Curcuma – 0, 5 tsp

Onion – 1 piece

Sea salt – 1, 5 tsp

Ground black pepper

Sprigs of rosemary – 2 pcs

Sprigs of thyme – 2 pcs

Instructions:

1. Take two tbsps of lemon juice. Pour juice in a large bowl, add two tablespoons of olive oil, 0,5 teaspoon of curcuma, sea salt and black pepper.

2. Marinade chicken thighs.

3. Slice two lemons and onion.

4. Take a large cast iron skillet, pour an olive oil and heat it

5. Put chicken thighs and fry on both sides for 8 minutes

6. Transfer fried thighs to a plate.

7. Put lemon and onion slices, herbs in the pan. Let stew for several minutes

8. Then pour 50 g of water into the pan and put the chicken back.

9. Stew chicken with mixture of lemon, herbs and onion for 10 minutes.

10. Flavorful Lebanese lemon chicken is ready!

11. Better serve with rice or cauliflower rice.

45. Paleo Chicken Bowl

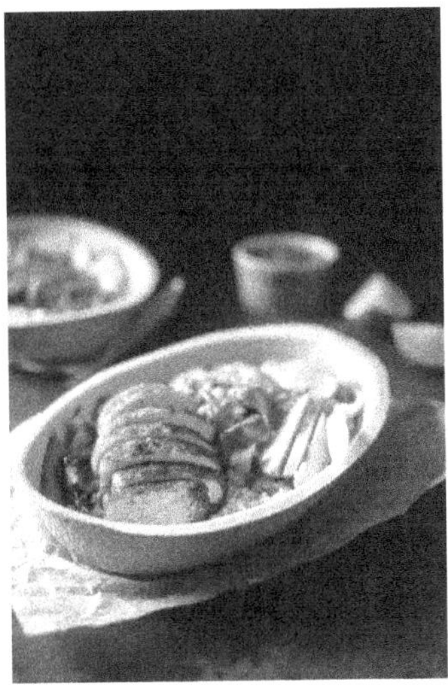

Ingredients:

Avocado – 2 pcs

Roasted peppers - 1 jar (335 g)

Garlic bulbet - 2 pcs

Chicken thighs – 500 g (boneless, skinless)

 Olive oil – 15ml

Red onion - one small

Sliced mushrooms – 300 g

Greens (any you like)

Salt and pepper

Instructions:

Make roasted pepper sauce

1. Take one avocado, drained roasted peppers, mashed garlic, salt and pepper. Put all ingredients into a kitchen machine. Mix until smooth and let the sauce cool.

Cook chicken

1. Do up chicken with salt and pepper. Take a large skillet, heat it and add olive oil. Fry chicken thighs brown on both sides.

2. While frying, peel and dice vegetables and greens.

3. Transfer the finished chicken to the dish.

4. Fry onion about 1-2 minutes, then add mushrooms and fry 2-3 minutes. Add greens and fry again about 1-2 minutes.

5. Divide the chicken into small portions and mix with fried vegetables.

6. Put into bowls.

8. Serve with roasted pepper sauce.

46. Paleo Baked Eggs in Tomatoes

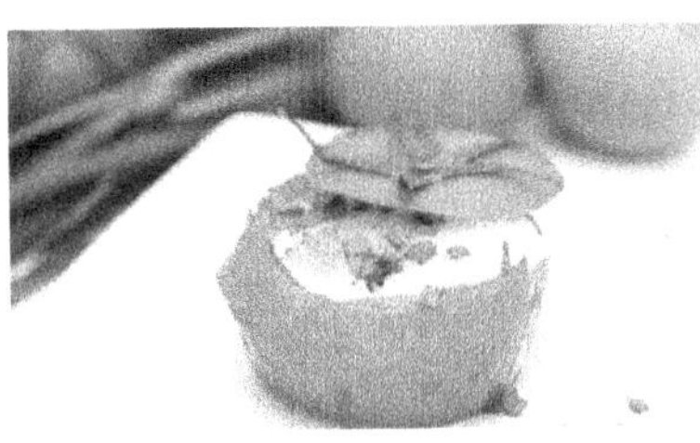

Ingredients:

Tomatoes in own juice – 1200 ml

Powdered garlic

Black pepper bacon – 6 slices

Organic eggs – 12 pcs

Chopped green onions – 3 pcs

Sea salt

Instructions:

1. Heat the oven to 180°C.

2. Pour tomatoes in own juice in a glass dish).

3. Mash the tomatoes. Season with powdered garlic and mix with the sliced black pepper bacon. Stir spicy tomato sauce thoroughly.

4. Break the eggs into this sauce (not scramble).

5. Drizzle with green and give relish to a dish (use pepper and salt.

6. Put it in the oven. Cook for 60 minutes.

7. Take ready baked eggs in tomatoes out of the oven.

8. Enjoy!

47. Indian Spiced Brussels & Carrots

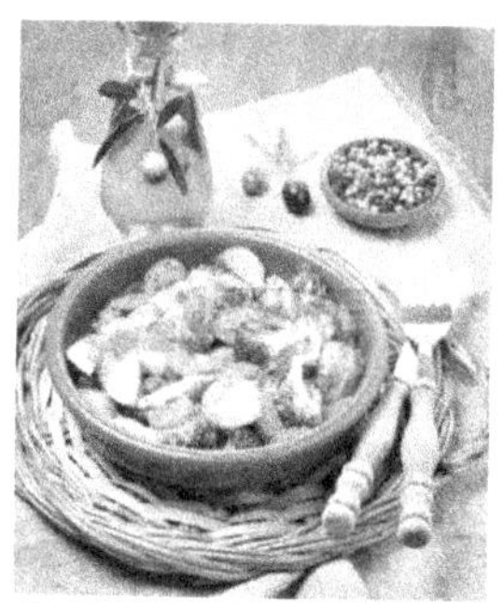

Ingredients:

Brussels sprouts – 1 kg

Carrots – 2 pcs , peeled & sliced

Garam masala

Sweet curry

Coriander

Coarse ground sea salt

Avocado oil

Instructions:

1. Prepare the oven. Heat it to 200°C.

2. Prepare the Brussels sprouts: chop the ends off, cut damaged outer peel

3. Cut the sprouts into equal parts. Spread these pieces into casserole dish

4. Add peeled and sliced carrot and season to taste. Sprinkle with avocado oil and mix thoroughly.

5. Put the dish to the oven and cook for 20 minutes.

6. Mix again and bake for 20-30 minutes until do brown.

7. Take the dish out of the oven.

8. Enjoy warm!

Paleo Smoothie Recipes

48. Very Berry Smoothie

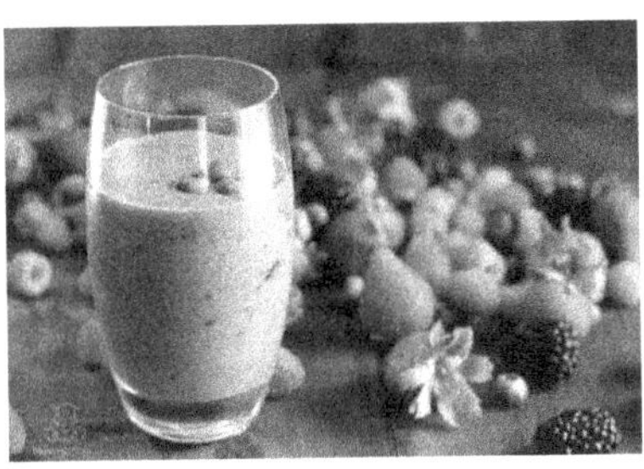

Ingredients:

Spinach - 2 cups

Mixed berries - 200-220 g

Frozen bananas – 1 piece

Peeled kiwi - 1 piece

Water - 480 ml

Instructions:

1. Blend spinach, berries, bananas, kiwi and water until smooth.

2. Enjoy your very berry smoothie.

49. Strawberry Banana Smoothie

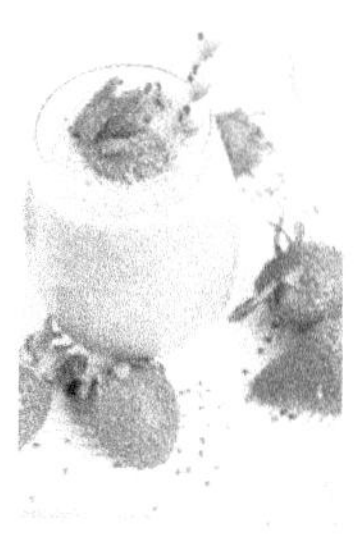

Ingredients:

Diced fresh strawberries – 100-170 g

Banana – 1 piece

Almond milk - 120 ml

Cube ice -200 g

Honey - 1/2 tbsp

Instructions:

1. Mix all of the components. Make a purée in blender until smooth.

2. If your smoothie is so thick – pour some almond milk to get your favorite consistency.

3. Put 0, 5 tbsp of honey (or more if necessary).

4. Drink immediately.

50. Mango Lime Smoothie

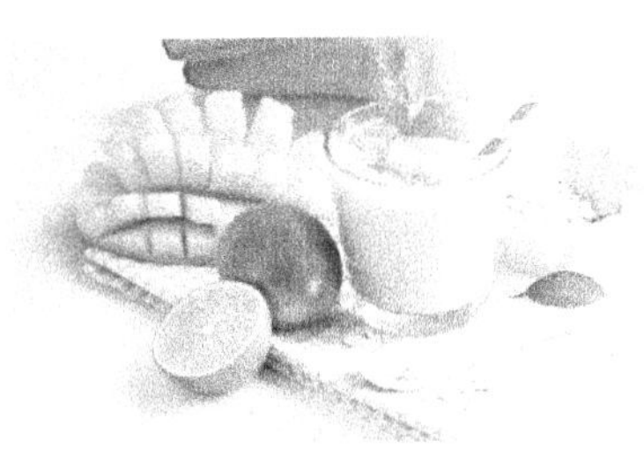

Ingredients:

Freshly squeezed lime juice - two tbsp

Spinach - 2 cups

Frozen mango – 250 g

Instructions:

1. Mix all of the components. Make a purée in blender until smooth

2. Help yourself!

51. Cinnamon Chia Smoothie

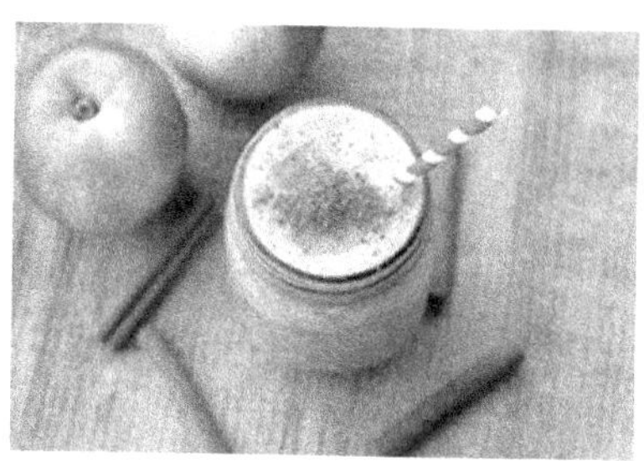

Ingredients:

Almond milk - 240 ml

Spinach - 1 cup

Peeled apple – 1 piece

Chia seeds – two tbsps

Maple syrup – one tbsp

Cinnamon - 0, 5 tbsp

Instructions:

1. Mix thoroughly all ingredients. Whisk until smooth.

2. Sprinkle smoothie with chia seeds

3. Enjoy this cinnamon chia smoothie!

52. Almond Cantaloupe Smoothie

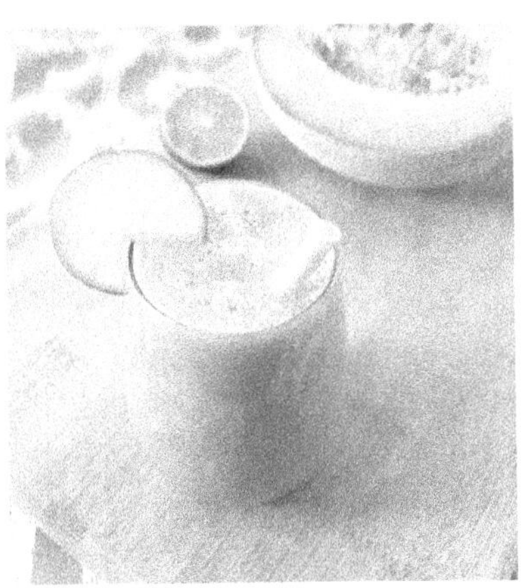

Ingredients:

Spinach – 250 g

Unsweetened almond milk – 240 ml

Mixed berries - 200-220 g

Sweet and peeled cantaloupe -   1/2

Water – 120 ml

Cube ice

Instructions:

1. Whisk all ingredients until smooth.

2. Pour in a glass with fresh smoothie several ice cubes.

3. Enjoy this tasty and healthy cool drink!

53. Paleo Desserts cookies recipes

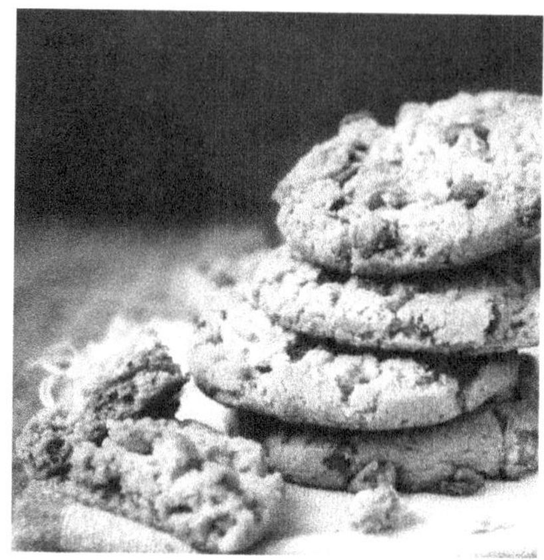

Ingredients:

 Almond butter - 225 g

Almonds- 100 g

Rich coconut milk – 240 ml

Unsweetened shredded coconut – 200 g

Fresh eggs – 3 pieces

A pinch of powered vanillin

Honey – two tbsp

Gel- molding frames - 1 package

Instructions:

1. Preheat oven to 400 F.

2. Combine all components.

3. Pour into gel- molding frames for muffins

4. Bake about 15 minutes.

54. Nut free banana bread

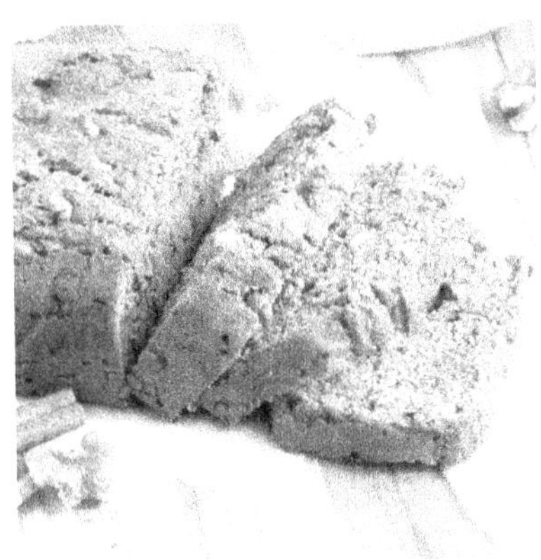

Ingredients:

Puree of one banana

Fresh eggs – 2 pcs

Sunflower seed butter peanut butter – 170 g

Maple syrup – 120 ml

Powered vanillin – one tbsp

Fresh lemon juice – 15 ml

Coconut oil – 30 ml

Starch (tapioca flour) - 70 g

Cinnamon - one tsp

Ground ginger (to taste)

Baking powder – one tsp

Tartar sauce – 5 ml

Ground nutmeg (to taste)

Sea salt

Instructions:

1. Preheat oven to 180 C.

2. Grease a loaf pan with 1 tbsp of coconut oil. Take a piece of wax paper and put it on the bottom of baking form. Grease wax paper with coconut oil too.

3. Take a bowl, mix together the tapioca flour, nutmeg, baking soda and add cinnamon, ginger, Tartar sauce and salt. Stir well.

4. Take a blender and mix puree of one banana, two eggs, 120 ml of maple syrup, 170 g of sunflower seeds butter, powered vanillin, lemon juice and coconut oil. Whisk carefully.

5. Add mixture of dry ingredients to the blender and beat until batter.

6. Remove the batter from the bowl and pour into the baking form.

7. Bake for 55-60 minutes until golden crust.

8. Let the dish to cool.

9. Slice as you like and enjoy!

55. Carrot Banana Muffins (for 12 servings)

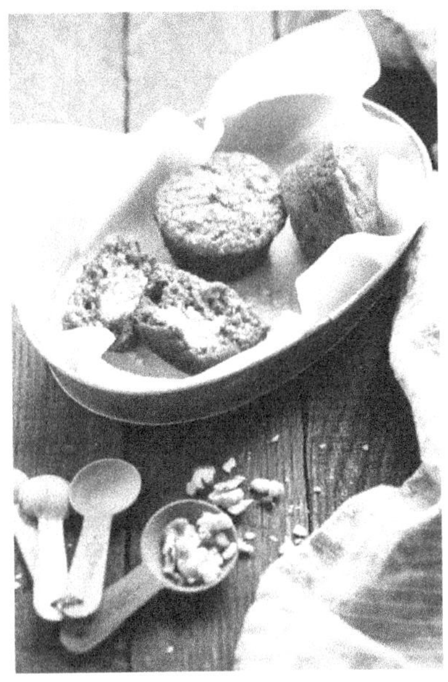

Ingredients:

Almond flour – 280 g

Baking powder – two tsp

Cinnamon - one tsp

Pitted dates – 100 g

Bananas – 3 pcs

Fresh eggs – 3 pcs

Cider vinegar – one tsp

Shredded carrot – 150 g

Finely chopped nuts (any kind of nut you like)

Gel- molding frames - 1 package

Melted coconut oil – 57 g

Sea salt

Instructions:

1. Heat oven to 180 C.

2. Take a deep, dry bowl to mix ingredients in accordance with the recipe (flour, a pinch of salt, baking powder and one teaspoon of cinnamon.

3. Combine bananas, eggs, dates, coconut oil, cider vinegar in a kitchen machine.

4. Join mixture from kitchen machine to dry components in the deep bowl. Whisk it thoroughly.

5. Add 150 g of shredded carrot and finely chopped nuts.

6. Move the batter from the bowl and pour into gel-molding frames for muffins.

7. Bake for 25 minute at 180 C

8. Here are your muffins - enjoy!

56. Fresh Zucchini Bread

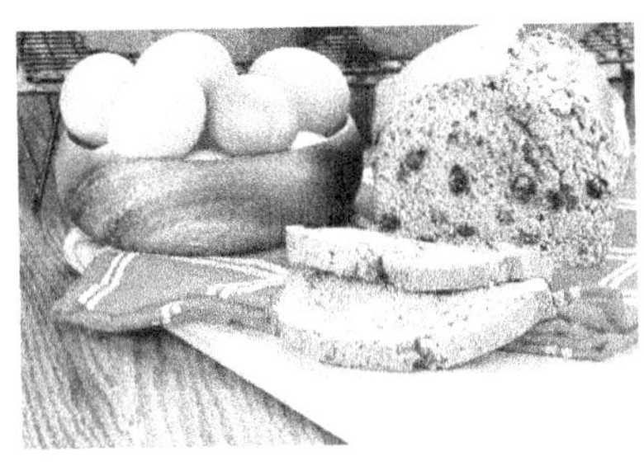

Ingredients: (per 8 servings)

One large grated zucchini

Kosher salt – 0, 5 tsp

Almond flour – 210 g

Baking powder – one tsp

Cinnamon - two tsps

Ground nutmeg (to taste)

Fresh eggs – 2 pcs

Melted coconut oil – 60 ml

Powered vanillin – one tbsp

Raw honey - 85 g

Instructions:

1. Heat oven to 180 C.

2. Grate one large zucchini. Add to this mass some salt and let sit for five minutes.

3. Pour away the excess water.

4. Combine dry components together. Mix well.

5. Take another bowl and blend eggs, powered vanillin, the coconut oil and honey. Spread this mixture into the dry components. Blend and add to zucchini.

6. Grease a cake tin with coconut oil, and pour the batter into it.

7. Bake about 35-45 minutes until do brown.

8. Let the zucchini bread to cool.

9. Slice it and enjoy!

57. Paleo Carrot Cake

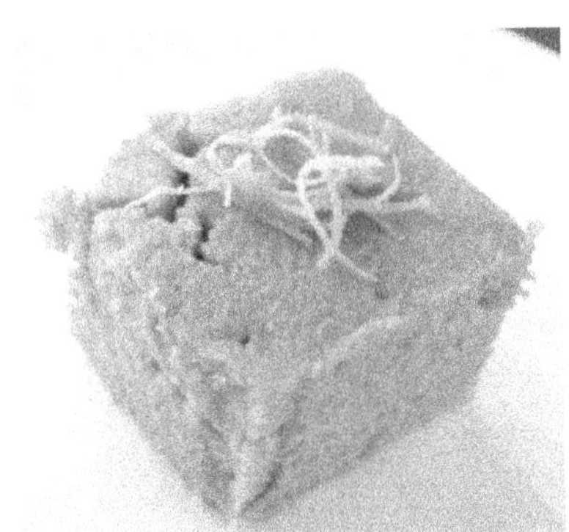

Ingredients:

Almond flour – 210 g

Coconut flour – 46 g

Arrowroot powder – 140 g

Cinnamon - one tbls

Baking powder – two tsp

Baking soda – one tsp

Maple syrup or honey – 170 g

Melted coconut oil – 3/4   cup

Powered vanillin – one tbsp

Orange zest – one tbsp

Grated carrot – three pcs(s)

Sea salt (to taste)

Ground ginger (to taste)

Ground nutmeg (to taste)

Eggs – 9 pcs

Glaze Ingredients:

Soaked cashews – 1 cup

Coconut oil - 13/4 cup

Coconut butter – 113 g

Fresh lemon juice – one tbsp

Maple syrup – 85 g

Powered vanillin – one tbsp vanilla

Cider vinegar – two tbsp.

Instructions:

Bake the cake.

1. Heat oven to 180 C. Grease baking case with coconut oil.

2. Mix dry ingredients.

3. Take another bowl, mix wet ingredients (except carrots) and blend.

4. Empty   dry mixture out of the dish and add to the wet. Stir well.

5. Put grated carrot. Pour the batter into prepared baking case.

6. Bake for 30-35 minutes until do brown.

7. Let the cake to cool down.

Make the glaze

1. Drain the cashews. Blend until creamy.

2. Put the rest ingredients for glaze and beat until creamy

3. Put the glaze over the cake.

4. Carrot cake is ready! Cut it and serve!

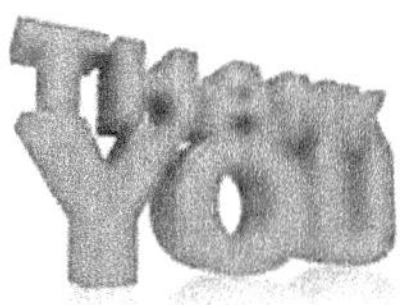

I am very happy that you have chosen this book and it's been a real pleasure writing it for you. My aim is to help as many readers as possible. So many of us are able to take new knowledge and use it to our lives with really useful and long lasting consequences and it is my desire that you have been able to take value from the information I have written.

Thank you for being with me during this recipe book and for reading it through to the end. I really hope that you have enjoyed all the recipes I provided you and that's why I appreciate your thoughts on my material so much. If you could take a couple of minutes to write a feedback, your views will help me to create more material that you find beneficial.

Thanks again for your attention. I really look forward to reading your review.

Stay Healthy!